THE ALZHEIMERS DISEASE

COOKBOOK FOR BEGINNERS

GEORGE ANDERSON

CHAPTER ONE

INTRODUCTION

Alzheimer's disease

Alzheimer's disease (AD) is a neurodegenerative disease that usually starts slowly and progressively worsens. It is the cause of 60–70% of cases of dementia. The most common early symptom is difficulty in remembering recent events. As the disease advances, symptoms can include problems with language, disorientation (including easily getting lost), mood swings, loss of motivation, self-neglect, and behavioral issues. As a person's condition declines, they often withdraw from family and society. Gradually, bodily functions are lost, ultimately leading to death. Although the speed of progression can vary, the typical life expectancy following diagnosis is three to nine years.

The cause of Alzheimer's disease is poorly understood. There are many environmental and genetic risk factors associated with its development.

The strongest genetic risk factor is from an allele of APOE. Other risk factors include a history of head injury, clinical depression, and high blood pressure. The disease process is largely associated with amyloid plaques, neurofibrillary tangles, and loss of neuronal connections in the brain. A probable diagnosis is based on the history of the illness and cognitive testing with medical imaging and blood tests to rule out other possible causes. Initial symptoms are often mistaken for normal aging. Examination of brain tissue is needed for a definite diagnosis, but this can only take place after death. Good nutrition, physical activity, and engaging socially are known to be of benefit generally in aging, and these may help in reducing the risk of cognitive decline and Alzheimer's; in 2019 clinical trials were underway to look at these possibilities. There are no medications or supplements that have been shown to decrease risk.

No treatments stop or reverse its progression, though some may temporarily improve symptoms. Affected people increasingly rely on others for assistance, often placing a burden on the caregiver. The pressures can include social, psychological, physical, and economic elements. Exercise programs may be beneficial with respect to activities of daily living and can potentially improve outcomes. Behavioral problems or psychosis due to dementia are often treated with antipsychotics, but this is not usually recommended, as there is little benefit and an increased risk of early death.

As of 2020, there were approximately 50 million people worldwide with Alzheimer's disease. It most often begins in people over 65 years of age, although up to 10% of cases are early-onset affecting those in their 30s to mid-60s. It affects about 6% of people 65 years and older, and women more often than men. The disease is named after German psychiatrist and pathologist Alois Alzheimer, who first described it in 1906. Alzheimer's financial burden on society is large, with an estimated global annual cost of US$1 trillion. Alzheimer's disease is currently ranked as the seventh leading cause of death in the United States.

SIGNS AND SYMPTOMS OF ALZHEIMER'S DISEASE

The course of Alzheimer's is generally described in three stages, with a progressive pattern of cognitive and functional impairment. The three stages are described as early or mild, middle or moderate, and late or severe. The disease is known to target the hippocampus which is associated with memory, and this is responsible for the first symptoms of memory impairment. As the disease progresses so does the degree of memory impairment.

First symptoms

The first symptoms are often mistakenly attributed to aging or stress. Detailed neuropsychological testing can reveal mild cognitive difficulties up to eight years before a person fulfills the clinical criteria for diagnosis of Alzheimer's disease. These early symptoms can affect the most complex activities of daily living. The most noticeable deficit is short term memory loss, which shows up as difficulty in remembering recently learned facts and inability to acquire new information.

Subtle problems with the executive functions of attentiveness, planning, flexibility, and abstract thinking, or impairments in semantic memory (memory of meanings, and concept relationships) can also be symptomatic of the early stages of Alzheimer's disease. Apathy and depression can be seen at this stage, with apathy remaining as the most persistent symptom throughout the course of the disease. Mild cognitive impairment (MCI) is often found to be a transitional stage between normal aging and dementia. MCI can present with a variety of symptoms, and when memory loss is the predominant symptom, it is termed amnestic MCI and is frequently seen as a prodromal stage of Alzheimer's disease. Amnestic MCI has a greater than 90% likelihood of being associated with Alzheimer's.

Early stage

In people with Alzheimer's disease, the increasing impairment of learning and memory eventually leads to a definitive diagnosis. In a small percentage, difficulties with language, executive functions, perception (agnosia), or execution of movements (apraxia) are more prominent than memory problems. Alzheimer's disease does not affect all memory capacities equally. Older memories of the person's life (episodic memory), facts learned (semantic memory), and implicit memory (the memory of the body on how to do things, such as using a fork to eat or how to drink from a glass) are affected to a lesser degree than new facts or memories.

Language problems are mainly characterised by a shrinking vocabulary and decreased word fluency, leading to a general impoverishment of oral and written language. In this stage, the person with Alzheimer's is usually capable of communicating basic ideas adequately. While performing fine motor tasks such as writing, drawing, or dressing, certain movement coordination and planning difficulties (apraxia) may be present, but they are commonly unnoticed. As the disease progresses, people with Alzheimer's disease can often continue to perform many tasks independently, but may need assistance or supervision with the most cognitively demanding activities.

Middle stage

Progressive deterioration eventually hinders independence, with subjects being unable to perform most common activities of daily living. Speech difficulties become evident due to an inability to recall vocabulary, which leads to frequent incorrect word substitutions (paraphasias). Reading and writing skills are also progressively lost. Complex motor sequences become less coordinated as time passes and Alzheimer's disease progresses, so the risk of falling increases. During this phase, memory problems worsen, and the person may fail to recognise close relatives. Long-term memory, which was previously intact, becomes impaired.

Behavioral and neuropsychiatric changes become more prevalent. Common manifestations are wandering, irritability and emotional lability, leading to crying, outbursts of unpremeditated aggression, or resistance to caregiving. Sundowning can also appear. Approximately 30% of people with Alzheimer's disease develop illusionary misidentifications and other delusional symptoms. Subjects also lose insight of their disease process and limitations (anosognosia). Urinary incontinence can develop. These symptoms create stress for relatives and caregivers, which can be reduced by moving the person from home care to other long-term care facilities.

Late stage

During the final stage, known as the late-stage or severe stage, there is complete dependence on caregivers. Language is reduced to simple phrases or even single words, eventually leading to complete loss of speech. Despite the loss of verbal language abilities, people can often understand and return emotional signals. Although aggressiveness can still be present, extreme apathy and exhaustion are much more common symptoms. People with Alzheimer's disease will ultimately not be able to perform even the simplest tasks independently; muscle mass and mobility deteriorates to the point where they are bedridden and unable to feed themselves. The cause of death is usually an external factor, such as infection of pressure ulcers or pneumonia, not the disease itself.

CAUSES OF ALZHEIMER'S DISEASE

Proteins fail to function normally. This disrupts the work of the brain cells affected and triggers a toxic cascade, ultimately leading to cell death and later brain shrinkage.

Alzheimer's disease is believed to occur when abnormal amounts of amyloid beta (Aβ), accumulating extracellularly as amyloid plaques and tau proteins, or intracellularly as neurofibrillary tangles, form in the brain, affecting neuronal functioning and connectivity, resulting in a progressive loss of brain function. This altered protein clearance ability is age-related, regulated by brain cholesterol, and associated with other neurodegenerative diseases.

Advances in brain imaging techniques allow researchers to see the development and spread of abnormal amyloid and tau proteins in the living brain, as well as changes in brain structure and function. Beta-amyloid is a fragment of a larger protein. When these fragments cluster together, a toxic effect appears on neurons and disrupt cell-to-cell communication. Larger deposits called amyloid plaques are thus further formed.

Tau proteins are responsible in neuron's internal support and transport system to carry nutrients and other essential materials. In Alzheimer's disease, the shape of tau proteins is altered and thus organize themselves into structures called neurofibrillary tangles. The tangles disrupt the transport system and are toxic to cells.

The cause for most Alzheimer's cases is still mostly unknown, except for 1–2% of cases where deterministic genetic differences have been identified. Several competing hypotheses attempt to explain the underlying cause; the two predominant hypotheses are the amyloid beta (Aβ) hypothesis and the cholinergic hypothesis.

The oldest hypothesis, on which most drug therapies are based, is the cholinergic hypothesis, which proposes that Alzheimer's disease is caused by reduced synthesis of the neurotransmitter acetylcholine. The loss of cholinergic neurons noted in the limbic system and cerebral cortex, is a key feature in the progression of Alzheimer's. The 1991 amyloid hypothesis postulated that extracellular amyloid beta (Aβ) deposits are the fundamental cause of the disease. Support for this postulate comes from the location of the gene for the amyloid precursor protein (APP) on chromosome 21, together with the fact that people with trisomy 21

(Down syndrome) who have an extra gene copy almost universally exhibit at least the earliest symptoms of Alzheimer's disease by 40 years of age. A specific isoform of apolipoprotein, APOE4, is a major genetic risk factor for Alzheimer's disease. While apolipoproteins enhance the breakdown of beta amyloid, some isoforms are not very effective at this task (such as APOE4), leading to excess amyloid buildup in the brain.

Genetic

Only 1–2% of Alzheimer's cases are inherited (autosomal dominant). These types are known as early onset familial Alzheimer's disease, can have a very early onset, and a faster rate of progression. Early onset familial Alzheimer's disease can be attributed to mutations in one of three genes: those encoding amyloid-beta precursor protein (APP) and presenilins PSEN1 and PSEN2. Most mutations in the APP and presenilin genes increase the production of a small protein called amyloid beta (Aβ)42, which is the main component of amyloid plaques. Some of the mutations merely alter the ratio between Aβ42 and the other major forms particularly Aβ40 without increasing Aβ42 levels. Two other genes associated with autosomal dominant Alzheimer's disease are ABCA7 and SORL1.

Most cases of Alzheimer's are not inherited and are termed sporadic Alzheimer's disease, in which environmental and genetic differences may act as risk factors. Most cases of sporadic Alzheimer's disease in contrast to familial Alzheimer's disease are late-onset Alzheimer's disease (LOAD) developing after the age of 65 years. Less than 5% of sporadic Alzheimer's disease have an earlier onset. The strongest genetic risk factor for sporadic Alzheimer's disease is APOEε4. APOEε4 is one of four alleles of apolipoprotein E (APOE). APOE plays a major role in lipid-binding proteins in lipoprotein particles and the epsilon4 allele disrupts this function. Between 40 and 80% of people with Alzheimer's disease possess at least one APOEε4 allele. The APOEε4 allele increases the risk of the disease by three times in heterozygotes and by 15 times in homozygotes. Like many human diseases, environmental effects and genetic modifiers result in incomplete penetrance. For example, certain Nigerian populations do not show the relationship between dose of APOEε4 and incidence or age-of-onset for Alzheimer's disease seen in other human populations.

Alleles in the TREM2 gene have been associated with a 3 to 5 times higher risk of developing Alzheimer's disease.

A Japanese pedigree of familial Alzheimer's disease was found to be associated with a deletion mutation of codon 693 of APP. This mutation and its association with Alzheimer's disease was first reported in 2008, and is known as the Osaka mutation. Only homozygotes with this mutation have an increased risk of developing Alzheimer's disease. This mutation accelerates $A\beta$ oligomerization but the proteins do not form the amyloid fibrils that aggregate into amyloid plaques, suggesting that it is the $A\beta$ oligomerization rather than the fibrils that may be the cause of this disease.

Mice expressing this mutation have all the usual pathologies of Alzheimer's disease.

Other hypotheses

The tau hypothesis proposes that tau protein abnormalities initiate the disease cascade. In this model, hyperphosphorylated tau begins to pair with other threads of tau as paired helical filaments. Eventually, they form neurofibrillary tangles inside nerve cell bodies. When this occurs, the microtubules disintegrate, destroying the structure of the cell's cytoskeleton which collapses the neuron's transport system.

A number of studies connect the misfolded amyloid beta and tau proteins associated with the pathology of Alzheimer's disease, as bringing about oxidative stress that leads to chronic inflammation. Sustained inflammation (neuroinflammation) is also a feature of other neurodegenerative diseases including Parkinson's disease, and ALS. Spirochete infections have also been linked to dementia. DNA damages accumulate in AD brains; reactive oxygen species may be the major source of this DNA damage.

Sleep disturbances are seen as a possible risk factor for inflammation in Alzheimer's disease. Sleep problems have been seen as a consequence of Alzheimer's disease but studies suggest that they may instead be a causal factor. Sleep disturbances are thought to be linked to persistent inflammation. The cellular homeostasis of biometals such as ionic copper, iron, and zinc is disrupted in Alzheimer's disease, though it remains unclear whether this is produced by or causes the changes in proteins. Smoking is a significant Alzheimer's disease risk factor. Systemic markers of the innate immune system are risk factors for late-onset Alzheimer's disease. Exposure to air pollution may be a contributing factor to the development of Alzheimer's disease.

One hypothesis posits that dysfunction of oligodendrocytes and their associated myelin during aging contributes to axon damage, which then causes amyloid production and tau hyper-phosphorylation as a side effect.

Retrogenesis is a medical hypothesis that just as the fetus goes through a process of neurodevelopment beginning with neurulation and ending with myelination, the brains of people with Alzheimer's disease go through a reverse neurodegeneration process starting with demyelination and death of axons (white matter) and ending with the death of grey matter. Likewise the hypothesis is, that as infants go through states of cognitive development, people with Alzheimer's disease go through the reverse process of progressive cognitive impairment.

The association with celiac disease is unclear, with a 2019 study finding no increase in dementia overall in those with CD, while a 2018 review found an association with several types of dementia including Alzheimer's disease.

PREVENTION OF ALZHEIMER'S DISEASE

There are no disease-modifying treatments available to cure Alzheimer's disease and because of this, AD research has focused on interventions to prevent the onset and progression. There is no evidence that supports any particular measure in preventing Alzheimer's, and studies of measures to prevent the onset or progression have produced inconsistent results. Epidemiological studies have proposed relationships between an individual's likelihood of developing AD and modifiable factors, such as medications, lifestyle, and diet. There are some challenges in determining whether interventions for Alzheimer's disease act as a primary prevention method, preventing the disease itself, or a secondary prevention method, identifying the early stages of the disease. These challenges include duration of intervention, different stages of disease at which intervention begins, and lack of standardization of inclusion criteria regarding biomarkers specific for Alzheimer's disease. Further research is needed to determine factors that can help prevent Alzheimer's disease.

Medication

Cardiovascular risk factors, such as hypercholesterolaemia, hypertension, diabetes, and smoking, are associated with a higher risk of onset and worsened course of AD. The use of statins to lower cholesterol may be of benefit in Alzheimer's. Antihypertensive and antidiabetic medications in individuals without overt cognitive impairment may decrease the risk of dementia by influencing cerebrovascular pathology. More research is needed to examine the relationship with Alzheimer's disease specifically; clarification of the direct role medications play versus other concurrent lifestyle changes (diet, exercise, smoking) is needed.

Depression is associated with an increased risk for Alzheimer's disease; management with antidepressants may provide a preventative measure.

Historically, long-term usage of non-steroidal anti-inflammatory drugs (NSAIDs) were thought to be associated with a reduced likelihood of developing Alzheimer's disease as it reduces inflammation; however, NSAIDs do not appear to be useful as a treatment. Additionally, because women have a higher incidence of Alzheimer's disease than men, it was once thought that estrogen deficiency during menopause was a risk factor. However, there is a lack of evidence to show that hormone replacement therapy (HRT) in menopause decreases risk of cognitive decline.

Lifestyle

Certain lifestyle activities, such as physical and cognitive exercises, higher education and occupational attainment, cigarette smoking, stress, sleep, and the management of other comorbidities including, diabetes and hypertension may affect the risk of developing Alzheimer's.

Physical exercise is associated with a decreased rate of dementia, and is effective in reducing symptom severity in those with AD. Memory and cognitive functions can be improved with aerobic exercises including brisk walking three times weekly for forty minutes. It may also induce neuroplasticity of the brain. Participating in mental exercises, such as reading, crossword puzzles, and chess have shown a potential to be preventative.

Higher education and occupational attainment, and participation in leisure activities, contribute to a reduced risk of developing Alzheimer's, or of delaying the onset of symptoms. This is compatible with the cognitive reserve theory, which states that some life experiences result in more efficient neural functioning providing the individual a cognitive reserve that delays the onset of dementia manifestations. Education delays the onset of Alzheimer's disease syndrome without changing the duration of the disease.

Cessation in smoking may reduce risk of developing Alzheimer's' disease, specifically in those who carry APOE $\varepsilon 4$ allele. The increased oxidative stress caused by smoking results in downstream inflammatory or neurodegenerative processes that may increase risk of developing AD. Avoidance of smoking, counseling and pharmacotherapies to quit smoking are used, and avoidance of environmental tobacco smoke is recommended.

Alzheimer's disease is associated with sleep disorders but the precise relationship is unclear. It was once thought that as people get older, the risk of developing sleep disorders and AD independently increase, but research is examining whether sleep disorders may increase the prevalence of AD. One theory is that the mechanisms to increase clearance of toxic substances, including Aβ, are active during sleep. With decreased sleep, a person is increasing Aβ production and decreasing Aβ clearance, resulting in Aβ accumulation. Receiving adequate sleep (approximately 7–8 hours) every night has become a potential lifestyle intervention to prevent the development of AD.

Stress is a risk factor for the development of Alzheimer's. The mechanism by which stress predisposes someone to development of Alzheimer's is unclear, but it is suggested that lifetime stressors may affect a person's epigenome, leading to an overexpression or under expression of specific genes. Although the relationship of stress and Alzheimer's is unclear, strategies to reduce stress and relax the mind may be helpful strategies in preventing the progression or Alzheimer's disease. Meditation, for instance, is a helpful lifestyle change to support cognition and well-being, though further research is needed to assess long-term effects.

MANAGEMENT OF ALZHEIMER'S DISEASE

There is no cure for Alzheimer's disease; available treatments offer relatively small symptomatic benefits but remain palliative in nature. Treatments can be divided into pharmaceutical, psychosocial, and caregiving.

Pharmaceutical

Medications used to treat the cognitive problems of Alzheimer's disease include: four acetylcholinesterase inhibitors (tacrine, rivastigmine, galantamine, and donepezil) and memantine, an NMDA receptor antagonist. The acetylcholinesterase inhibitors are intended for those with mild to severe Alzheimer's, whereas memantine is intended for those with moderate or severe Alzheimer's disease. The benefit from their use is small.

Reduction in the activity of the cholinergic neurons is a well-known feature of Alzheimer's disease. Acetylcholinesterase inhibitors are employed to reduce the rate at which acetylcholine (ACh) is broken down, thereby increasing the concentration of ACh in the brain and combating the loss of ACh caused by the death of cholinergic neurons. There is evidence for the efficacy of these medications in mild to moderate Alzheimer's disease, and some evidence for their use in the advanced stage. The use of these drugs in mild cognitive impairment has not shown any effect in a delay of the onset of Alzheimer's disease. The most common side effects are nausea and vomiting, both of which are linked to cholinergic excess. These side effects arise in approximately 10–20% of users, are mild to moderate in severity, and can be managed by slowly adjusting medication doses. Less common secondary effects include muscle cramps, decreased heart rate (bradycardia), decreased appetite and weight, and increased gastric acid production.

Glutamate is an excitatory neurotransmitter of the nervous system, although excessive amounts in the brain can lead to cell death through a process called excitotoxicity which consists of the overstimulation of glutamate receptors. Excitotoxicity occurs not only in Alzheimer's disease, but also in other neurological diseases such as Parkinson's disease and multiple sclerosis. Memantine is a noncompetitive NMDA receptor antagonist first used as an anti-influenza agent. It acts on the glutamatergic system by blocking NMDA receptors and inhibiting their overstimulation by glutamate.

Memantine has been shown to have a small benefit in the treatment of moderate to severe Alzheimer's disease. Reported adverse events with memantine are infrequent and mild, including hallucinations, confusion, dizziness, headache and fatigue. The combination of memantine and donepezil has been shown to be "of statistically significant but clinically marginal effectiveness".

An extract of Ginkgo biloba known as EGb 761 has been widely used for treating Alzheimer's and other neuropsychiatric disorders. Its use is approved throughout Europe. The World Federation of Biological Psychiatry guidelines lists EGb 761 with the same weight of evidence (level B) given to acetylcholinesterase inhibitors, and memantine. EGb 761 is the only one that showed improvement of symptoms in both Alzheimer's disease and vascular dementia. EGb 761 is seen as being able to play an important role either on its own or as an add-on particularly when other therapies prove ineffective. EGb 761 is seen to be neuroprotective; it is a free radical scavenger, improves mitochondrial function, and modulates serotonin and dopamine levels. Many studies of its use in mild to moderate dementia have shown it to significantly improve cognitive function, activities of daily living, and neuropsychiatric symptoms. However, its use has not been shown to prevent the progression to dementia.

Atypical antipsychotics are modestly useful in reducing aggression and psychosis in people with Alzheimer's disease, but their advantages are offset by serious adverse effects, such as stroke, movement difficulties or cognitive decline. When used in the long-term, they have been shown to associate with increased mortality. Stopping antipsychotic use in this group of people appears to be safe.

Psychosocial

Psychosocial interventions are used as an adjunct to pharmaceutical treatment and can be classified within behavior-, emotion-, cognition- or stimulation-oriented approaches.

Behavioral interventions attempt to identify and reduce the antecedents and consequences of problem behaviors. This approach has not shown success in improving overall functioning, but can help to reduce some specific problem behaviors, such as incontinence. There is a lack of high quality data on the effectiveness of these techniques in other behavior problems such as wandering. Music therapy is effective in reducing behavioral and psychological symptoms.

Emotion-oriented interventions include reminiscence therapy, validation therapy, supportive psychotherapy, sensory integration, also called snoezelen, and simulated presence therapy. A Cochrane review has found no evidence that this is effective. Reminiscence therapy (RT) involves the discussion of past experiences individually or in group, many times with the aid of photographs, household items, music and sound recordings, or other familiar items from the past. A 2018 review of the effectiveness of RT found that effects were inconsistent, small in size and of doubtful clinical significance, and varied by setting. Simulated presence therapy (SPT) is based on attachment theories and involves playing a recording with voices of the closest relatives of the person with Alzheimer's disease. There is partial evidence indicating that SPT may reduce challenging behaviors.

The aim of cognition-oriented treatments, which include reality orientation and cognitive retraining, is the reduction of cognitive deficits. Reality orientation consists of the presentation of information about time, place, or person to ease the understanding of the person about its surroundings and his or her place in them. On the other hand, cognitive retraining tries to improve impaired capacities by exercising mental abilities. Both have shown some efficacy improving cognitive capacities.

Stimulation-oriented treatments include art, music and pet therapies, exercise, and any other kind of recreational activities. Stimulation has modest support for improving behavior, mood, and, to a lesser extent, function. Nevertheless, as important as these effects are, the main support for the use of stimulation therapies is the change in the person's routine.

Caregiving

Since Alzheimer's has no cure and it gradually renders people incapable of tending to their own needs, caregiving is essentially the treatment and must be carefully managed over the course of the disease.

During the early and moderate stages, modifications to the living environment and lifestyle can increase safety and reduce caretaker burden. Examples of such modifications are the adherence to simplified routines, the placing of safety locks, the labeling of household items to cue the person with the disease or the use of modified daily life objects. If eating becomes problematic, food will need to be prepared in smaller pieces or even puréed. When swallowing difficulties arise, the use of feeding tubes may be required. In such cases, the medical efficacy and ethics of continuing feeding is an important consideration of the caregivers and family members. The use of physical restraints is rarely indicated in any stage of the disease, although there are situations when they are necessary to prevent harm to the person with Alzheimer's disease or their caregivers.

During the final stages of the disease, treatment is centred on relieving discomfort until death, often with the help of hospice.

Diet

Diet may be a modifiable risk factor for the development of Alzheimer's disease. The Mediterranean diet, and the DASH diet are both associated with less cognitive decline. A different approach has been to incorporate elements of both of these diets into one known as the MIND diet. Studies of individual dietary components, minerals and supplements are conflicting as to whether they prevent AD or cognitive decline.

CHAPTER TWO

ALZHEIMER'S DISEASE RECIPES

Here are some important recipes you should feed people with Alzheimer's disease, each of the recipes in this book is explained in details;

Oven-Poached Salmon Fillets

Ingredients

- 1 pound salmon fillet, cut into 4 portions, skin removed, if desired

- 2 tablespoons dry white wine

- ¼ teaspoon salt

- Freshly ground pepper, to taste

- 2 tablespoons finely chopped shallot, (1 medium)

- Lemon wedges, for garnish

Directions

- Step 1

Preheat oven to 425 degrees F. Coat a 9-inch glass pie pan or an 8-inch glass baking dish with cooking spray.

- Step 2

Place salmon, skin-side (or skinned-side) down, in the prepared pan. Sprinkle with wine. Season with salt and pepper, then sprinkle with shallots. Cover with foil and bake until opaque in the center and starting to flake, 15 to 25 minutes, depending on thickness.

- Step 3

When the salmon is ready, transfer to dinner plates. Spoon any liquid remaining in the pan over the salmon and serve with lemon wedges.

Mac & Cheese with Collards

Ingredients

- 8 ounces whole-wheat elbow noodles (about 2 cups)

- 4 cups chopped collard greens

- 1 ¾ cups low-fat milk, divided

- 3 tablespoons all-purpose flour

- ½ teaspoon salt

- ¼ teaspoon ground pepper

- 1 cup shredded extra-sharp Cheddar cheese

- 2 ounces reduced-fat cream cheese

- 2 teaspoons white-wine vinegar

- ¼ cup panko breadcrumbs, preferably whole-wheat

- 1 tablespoon extra-virgin olive oil

- ½ teaspoon paprika

Directions

- Step 1

Bring a large pot of water to a boil. Add pasta and collards and cook according to the pasta package directions. Drain.

- Step 2

Meanwhile, heat 1 1/2 cups milk in a large broiler-safe skillet over medium-high heat until just simmering. Whisk the remaining 1/4 cup milk, flour, salt and pepper in a small bowl until combined. Add the flour mixture to the simmering milk; reduce heat to medium-low and cook, whisking constantly, until thickened, 1 to 2 minutes. Remove from heat and whisk in Cheddar, cream cheese and vinegar until the cheese is melted. Stir the pasta and collards into the sauce.

- Step 3

Position rack in upper third of oven; preheat broiler to high.

- Step 4

Combine breadcrumbs, oil and paprika in a small bowl. Sprinkle over the pasta. Broil until golden brown, 1 to 3 minutes.

Grilled Salmon and Peaches with Basil-Pistachio Gremolata

Ingredients

- 1 teaspoon ground cumin

- 1 teaspoon chili powder

- 1 teaspoon brown sugar

- 1 teaspoon kosher salt, divided

- ½ teaspoon garlic powder

- ¼ teaspoon ground red pepper

- 1 (1 1/2 pound) salmon fillet, skin-on

- Cooking spray

- 1 small red onion (about 9 ounces)

- 2 large peaches, slightly firm

- 2 tablespoons olive oil

- ¼ cup chopped dry-roasted pistachios

- ¼ cup chopped fresh basil

- 2 teaspoons grated lemon zest

Directions

- Step 1

Prepare grill for indirect grilling: Heat one side of a gas grill to medium-high (400 degrees F), or push hot coals to one side of a charcoal grill. Maintain temperature at about 400 degrees F.

- Step 2

Combine cumin, chili powder, sugar, 3/4 teaspoon salt, garlic powder, and red pepper; rub evenly over flesh side of salmon.

- Step 3

Cut onion into 8 wedges, leaving root end intact. Cut each peach in half, remove pit, and cut each half into 4 wedges (16 wedges total). Place onion and peach wedges in a medium bowl; drizzle with oil, and toss gently to coat.

- Step 4

Arrange salmon over hot coals on oiled grill rack (over direct heat); close lid and grill until skin becomes crisp and lightly browned, 4 to 5 minutes. Move salmon to unheated side of grill for indirect grilling: On a gas grill, turn off burners under salmon and turn on burners on the other side of grill; on charcoal grill, carefully rotate grill rack using oven mitts so that salmon is over unheated side of grill. Arrange onion and peach wedges over hot coals on oiled grill rack (over direct heat). Close lid and grill until salmon flakes when tested with a fork and onion and peach wedges are well marked, about 4 to 5 minutes for salmon (no need to flip) and 1 to 2 minutes per side for onions and peaches. Remove from grill; sprinkle onion with remaining 1/4 teaspoon salt. Arrange salmon, peach wedges, and onion wedges on a platter.

- Step 5

Combine pistachios, basil, and lemon zest. Sprinkle evenly over platter.

Chicken & Veggie Fajitas

Ingredients

- 2 teaspoons canola or olive oil

- 1 pound boneless, skinless chicken thighs, trimmed and cut into strips

- 4 cups thinly sliced vegetables, such as onions, bell peppers, zucchini, and/or mushrooms (14 oz.)

- 1 ¼ teaspoons chili powder

- ¼ teaspoon salt

- 4 8-inch whole-wheat tortillas

- ½ cup prepared guacamole

- ½ cup nonfat plain Greek yogurt

- 1 lime, cut into wedges

- ¼ cup cilantro leaves (Optional)

Directions

- Step 1

Heat oil in a large wok or cast-iron or other stick-resistant skillet (not Teflon-based nonstick, see Tip) over high heat. Add chicken, vegetables, chili powder, and salt; cook, tossing with tongs occasionally, until the chicken is cooked through and the vegetables begin to brown, about 7 minutes.

• Step 2

Meanwhile, stack tortillas and wrap in a barely damp, clean kitchen towel (or paper towel). Microwave on High for 30 to 45 seconds.

• Step 3

Divide the chicken-and-vegetable mixture among the tortillas. Top each with 2 Tbsp. guacamole and 2 Tbsp. yogurt. Serve with lime wedges and garnish with cilantro if desired.

Almond-&-Lemon-Crusted Fish with Spinach

Ingredients

- Zest and juice of 1 lemon, divided

- ½ cup sliced almonds, coarsely chopped

- 1 tablespoon finely chopped fresh dill or 1 teaspoon dried

- 1 tablespoon plus 2 teaspoons extra-virgin olive oil, divided

- 1 teaspoon kosher salt, divided

- Freshly ground pepper to taste

- 1 1/4 pounds cod (see Tip) or halibut, cut into 4 portions

- 4 teaspoons Dijon mustard

- 2 cloves garlic, slivered

- 1 pound baby spinach

- Lemon wedges for garnish

Directions

- Step 1

Preheat oven to 400 degrees F. Coat a rimmed baking sheet with cooking spray.

- Step 2

Combine lemon zest, almonds, dill, 1 tablespoon oil, 1/2 teaspoon salt and pepper in a small bowl. Place fish on the prepared baking sheet and spread each portion with 1 teaspoon mustard. Divide the almond mixture among the portions, pressing it onto the mustard.

- Step 3

Bake the fish until opaque in the center, about 7 to 9 minutes, depending on thickness.

- Step 4

Meanwhile, heat the remaining 2 teaspoons oil in a Dutch oven over medium heat. Add garlic and cook, stirring, until fragrant but not brown, about 30 seconds. Stir in spinach, lemon juice and the remaining 1/2 teaspoon salt; season with pepper. Cook, stirring often, until the spinach is just wilted, 2 to 4 minutes. Cover to keep warm. Serve the fish with the spinach and lemon wedges, if desired.

Soup Beans

Ingredients

- 1 pound pinto, yellow-eyed or other dried beans, sorted and rinsed (2 1/2 cups)

- 12 cups water

- 8 ounces finely diced ham, (about 1 1/2 cups)

- 1 medium onion, peeled

- 1 clove garlic, peeled

- ½ teaspoon salt

- 1 teaspoon freshly ground pepper

- ¼ teaspoon crushed red pepper

Directions

- Step 1

Place beans, water, ham, onion, garlic, salt, pepper and crushed red pepper in a large Dutch oven; bring to a boil. Reduce heat and simmer, stirring occasionally, until the beans are very tender and beginning to burst, 1 1/2 to 2 hours. If necessary, add an additional 1/2 to 1 cup water while simmering to keep the beans just submerged in cooking liquid.

- Step 2

Remove from the heat; discard the onion and garlic. Transfer 2 cups of the beans to a medium bowl and coarsely mash with a fork or potato masher. Return the mashed beans to the pot; stir to combine.

Chickpea Pasta with Lemony-Parsley Pesto

Ingredients

* 4 ounces chickpea penne or other penne pasta (about 1 1/4 cups dry)

* 1 bunch flat-leaf parsley (about 4 cups lightly packed), plus more for garnish

* 3 cloves garlic

* ⅓ cup extra-virgin olive oil

* 1 teaspoon lemon zest

* 2 tablespoons lemon juice

* ½ teaspoon kosher salt

* ¼ teaspoon ground black pepper

* 1 1/2 cups roasted root vegetables (see associated recipe)

Directions

* Step 1

Cook pasta according to package directions. Drain well.

- Step 2

Meanwhile, combine parsley and garlic in a food processor and pulse until uniformly chopped, about 10 times. Add oil, lemon juice, salt and pepper and puree until just combined, about 15 seconds; it should be chunky.

- Step 3

Microwave roasted root vegetables in a microwave-safe bowl until heated through, about 1 minute. (Alternatively, heat 1 teaspoon extra-virgin olive oil in a large skillet over medium-high heat. Add vegetables and cook, stirring often, until heated through, 2 to 4 minutes.)

- Step 4

Toss the hot pasta with the pesto, the vegetables and lemon zest. Garnish with parsley, if desired.

25-Minute Chicken & Veggie Enchiladas

Ingredients

- 2 tablespoons canola oil

- 1 ½ cups chopped zucchini

- 1 ½ cups chopped yellow squash

- ½ cup chopped yellow onion

- 1 teaspoon minced garlic

- 1 ½ cups shredded, cooked chicken breast (about 4 1/2 oz.)

- ½ cup shredded, cooked chicken thigh (about 1 1/2 oz.)

- ⅝ teaspoon kosher salt

- ½ teaspoon black pepper

- 4 ounces Monterey Jack cheese, shredded (about 1 cup), divided

- 8 (6 inch) corn tortillas

- Cooking spray

- ½ cup bottled salsa verde

- Fresh cilantro leaves

Directions

- Step 1

Preheat oven to broil with rack 5 to 6 inches from heat. Heat oil in a large nonstick skillet over medium-high. Add zucchini, squash, and onion, and cook, stirring often, until vegetables are tender and just beginning to brown, about 10 minutes. Add garlic, and cook 1 more minute. Add chicken, salt, pepper, and 3/4 cup of the cheese; stir to combine. Cook until hot and cheese melts, about 1 minute. Remove from heat, and cover to keep warm.

- Step 2

Warm tortillas according to package directions. Place about 1/3 cup of chicken mixture in center of each tortilla; fold tortilla around filling, and place, seam side down, in a lightly greased (with cooking spray) 11- x 7-inch (or a 2-quart) broiler-safe baking dish. Pour salsa over enchiladas, and sprinkle with remaining 1/4 cup cheese. Broil in preheated oven until hot and bubbly, about 1 1/2 minutes. Garnish with cilantro.

Vegetarian Gumbo

Ingredients

- ½ cup all-purpose flour

- ⅓ cup extra-virgin olive oil

- 1 small butternut squash, peeled, seeded and cubed (3/4- to 1-inch)

- 2 cups chopped yellow onions

- 2 cups chopped poblano peppers

- 1 cup chopped celery

- 8 cups low-sodium vegetable broth

- 1 (28 ounce) can whole plum tomatoes, drained and crushed

- 1 ¾ teaspoons salt

- 3 cups fresh okra, trimmed and sliced (3/4-inch)

- 3 cups chopped zucchini

- 2 (15 ounce) cans no-salt-added pinto beans, rinsed

- 2 tablespoons hot sauce

- 1 tablespoon red-wine vinegar

- ½ teaspoon ground pepper

- 4 cups cooked brown rice, warmed

Directions

- Step 1

Whisk flour and oil in a 7-quart pot. Cook over medium heat, stirring frequently, until the mixture is deeply browned (the color of milk chocolate), 10 to 12 minutes. Add squash, onions, poblanos and celery; cook, stirring occasionally, until the vegetables are well coated and warmed through, about 5 minutes. Stir in broth, crushed tomatoes and salt; bring the mixture to a boil over high heat. Stir in okra; reduce heat to medium-high and simmer for

5 minutes. Stir in zucchini and beans; simmer until the squash is tender, about 5 minutes. Stir in hot sauce, vinegar and pepper. Serve over rice.

Almond-Thyme-Crusted Mahi Mahi with Lemon Chardonnay Sauce

Ingredients

- Nonstick cooking spray

- 4 4- to 5- ounce fresh or frozen mahi mahi fillets

- 1 egg white, lightly beaten

- 1 tablespoon water

- ⅓ cup sliced almonds, coarsely broken

- 2 tablespoons fine dry bread crumbs

- 1 tablespoon snipped fresh thyme

- ¼ teaspoon salt

- 1 tablespoon light butter with canola oil

- 1 tablespoon finely chopped shallot

- 1 ½ teaspoons all-purpose flour

- ⅛ teaspoon salt

- Dash black pepper

- ½ cup dry white wine, such as Chardonnay

- 1 tablespoon lemon juice

- ½ teaspoon snipped fresh thyme

- 1 teaspoon Snipped fresh thyme

Directions

- Step 1

Preheat oven to 450 degrees F. Line a baking sheet with foil. Coat foil with cooking spray; set aside. Thaw fish, if frozen. Rinse fish; pat dry with paper towels. Measure thickness of fish; set aside.

- Step 2

In a shallow dish, combine egg white and the water. In a second shallow dish, combine almonds, bread crumbs, the 1 tablespoon thyme, and the 1/4 teaspoon salt. Dip fillets in egg white mixture, turning to coat. Dip in almond mixture, turning to coat evenly.

- Step 3

Place fish on prepared baking sheet. Sprinkle any remaining almond mixture over fish. Coat fish with cooking spray. Bake 4 to 6 minutes per 1/2-inch thickness or until fish begins to flake easily when tested with a fork.

- Step 4

Meanwhile, in a small saucepan melt butter over medium heat. Add shallot; cook 3 minutes, stirring occasionally. Add flour, the 1/8 teaspoon salt, and the pepper, stirring until flour is coated. Add white wine and lemon juice all at once. Cook and stir until thickened and bubbly. Cook and stir 1 minute more. Remove from heat. Stir in the 1/2 teaspoon thyme. Drizzle sauce over fish to serve. If desired, garnish with additional snipped thyme.

Chicken Thighs with Couscous & Kale

Ingredients

- 1 ½ teaspoons dried thyme

- 1 ½ teaspoons ground cumin

- ¼ teaspoon salt

- ¼ teaspoon pepper

- 4 large boneless, skinless chicken thighs (about 1 1/4 pounds), trimmed

- 2 tablespoons extra-virgin olive oil, divided

- 1 medium onion, halved and sliced

- 1 cup Israeli couscous

- 2 cloves garlic, minced

- 4 cups very thinly sliced kale

- 2 cups reduced-sodium chicken broth

Directions

- Step 1

Combine thyme, cumin, salt and pepper in a small bowl. Sprinkle both sides of chicken with half of the spice mixture.

- Step 2

Heat 1 tablespoon oil in a large, heavy skillet, such as cast-iron, over medium-high heat. Add chicken and cook until golden brown, 2 to 3 minutes per side. Transfer to a plate.

- Step 3

Add the remaining 1 tablespoon oil and onion to the pan; cook, stirring frequently, until beginning to soften, 2 to 4 minutes. Stir in couscous and garlic; cook, stirring frequently, until the couscous is lightly toasted, 1 to 2 minutes. Add kale and the remaining spice mixture; cook, stirring, until the kale begins to wilt, 1 to 2 minutes.

- Step 4

Pour in broth and any accumulated juice from the chicken, then nestle the chicken into the couscous. Reduce the heat to medium-low, cover and cook until the chicken is cooked through and the couscous is tender, 10 to 12 minutes.

Escarole & White Bean Salad with Swordfish

Ingredients

- ¼ cup extra-virgin olive oil

- 2 tablespoons lemon juice

- 1 teaspoon Dijon mustard

- ½ teaspoon salt, divided

- ½ teaspoon ground pepper, divided

- 1 15-ounce can white beans, rinsed

- 2 10-ounce swordfish steaks

- 1 teaspoon herbes de Provence

- 12 cups chopped escarole

- ¼ cup very thinly sliced red onion

Directions

- Step 1

Position rack in upper third of oven; preheat broiler to high. Line a broiler-safe pan with foil.

- Step 2

Whisk oil, lemon juice, mustard and 1/4 teaspoon each salt and pepper in a large bowl. Transfer 2 tablespoons of the dressing to a small bowl. Add beans to the dressing in the large bowl and toss to combine.

- Step 3

Cut each swordfish steak in half so you have 4 equal portions; sprinkle with herbes de Provence and the remaining 1/4 teaspoon each salt and pepper. Place the fish on the prepared pan and broil on the upper rack until it just barely flakes when pressed with a knife, 8 to 10 minutes.

- Step 4

Toss escarole and onion with the beans. Serve the salad with the swordfish, drizzled with the reserved 2 tablespoons dressing.

Rainbow Grain Bowl with Cashew Tahini Sauce

Ingredients

- ¾ cup unsalted cashews

- ½ cup water

- ¼ cup packed parsley leaves

- 1 tablespoon lemon juice or cider vinegar

- 1 tablespoon extra-virgin olive oil

- ½ teaspoon reduced-sodium tamari or soy sauce (see Tip)

- ¼ teaspoon salt

- ½ cup cooked lentils

- ½ cup cooked quinoa

- ½ cup shredded red cabbage

- ¼ cup grated raw beet

- ¼ cup chopped bell pepper

- ¼ cup grated carrot

- ¼ cup sliced cucumber

- 1 tablespoon Toasted chopped cashews for garnish

Directions

- Step 1

Blend cashews, water, parsley, lemon juice (or vinegar), oil, tamari (or soy sauce) and salt in a blender until smooth.

- Step 2

Place lentils and quinoa in the center of a shallow serving bowl. Top with cabbage, beet, pepper, carrot and cucumber. Spoon 2 tablespoons of the cashew sauce over the top (save extra sauce for another use). Garnish with cashews, if desired.

Shrimp & Cheddar Grits

Ingredients

- 1 14-ounce can reduced-sodium chicken broth

- 1 ½ cups water

- 3/4 cup quick grits, (not instant) (see Shopping Tip)

- ½ teaspoon freshly ground pepper, divided

- ¾ cup extra-sharp or sharp Cheddar cheese

- 1 pound peeled and deveined raw shrimp, (16-20 per pound; see Shopping Tip)

- 1 bunch scallions, trimmed and cut into 1-inch pieces

- 1 tablespoon extra-virgin olive oil

- ¼ teaspoon garlic powder

- ⅛ teaspoon salt

Directions

- Step 1

Position rack in upper third of oven; preheat broiler.

- Step 2

Bring broth and water to a boil in a large saucepan over medium-high heat. Whisk in grits and 1/4 teaspoon pepper. Reduce heat to medium-low, cover and cook, stirring occasionally, until thickened, 5 to 7 minutes. Remove from heat and stir in cheese. Cover to keep warm.

- Step 3

Meanwhile, toss shrimp, scallions, oil, garlic powder, the remaining 1/4 teaspoon pepper and salt in a medium bowl. Transfer to a rimmed baking sheet. Broil, stirring once, until the shrimp are pink and just cooked through, 5 to 6 minutes. Serve the grits topped with the broiled shrimp and scallions.

Pistachio-Crusted Chicken with Warm Barley Salad

Ingredients

- Olive oil or canola oil cooking spray

- 2 cups water plus 1 tablespoon, divided

- 1 cup quick barley

- 1 cup salted shelled pistachios, divided

- ½ cup whole-wheat panko breadcrumbs

- 1 teaspoon orange zest

- ½ teaspoon garlic powder

- 1 large egg white

- 2 (8 ounce) boneless, skinless chicken breasts, trimmed and cut in half crosswise

- ½ teaspoon salt, divided

- 2 tablespoons extra-virgin olive oil

- 1 cup cherry tomatoes, halved

- 1 tablespoon white-wine vinegar

- 1 cup chopped fresh parsley

Directions

- Step 1

Preheat oven to 450 degrees F. Coat a wire rack with cooking spray and place on a foil-lined baking sheet.

- Step 2

Bring 2 cups water and barley to a boil in a small saucepan. Reduce heat, cover and simmer until tender, 10 to 12 minutes. Set aside.

- Step 3

Meanwhile, pulse 3/4 cup pistachios, breadcrumbs, orange zest and garlic powder in a food processor until the pistachios are coarsely chopped. Transfer to a shallow dish. Whisk egg white and the remaining 1 tablespoon water in another shallow dish.

- Step 4

Place chicken between 2 pieces of plastic wrap. Pound with the smooth side of a meat mallet or heavy saucepan to an even 1/2-inch thickness. Sprinkle the chicken with 1/4 teaspoon salt, coat with the egg mixture and dredge in the pistachio mixture, patting to adhere. Place on the prepared rack. Coat both sides of the chicken with cooking spray.

• Step 5

Bake the chicken until an instant-read thermometer inserted in the thickest part registers 165 degrees F, about 15 minutes.

• Step 6

Heat oil in a large skillet over medium heat. Add tomatoes and vinegar. Cook until the tomatoes just start to collapse, about 1 minute. Remove from heat.

• Step 7

Drain the barley, if necessary, and stir into the tomatoes along with the remaining 1/4 cup pistachios, 1/4 teaspoon salt and parsley. Serve with the chicken.

Salmon with Roasted Red Pepper Quinoa Salad

Ingredients

- 3 tablespoons extra-virgin olive oil, divided

- 1 ¼ pounds skin-on salmon, preferably wild, cut into 4 portions

- ½ teaspoon salt, divided

- ½ teaspoon ground pepper, divided

- 2 tablespoons red-wine vinegar

- 1 clove garlic, grated

- 2 cups cooked quinoa (see Tip)

- 1 cup chopped roasted red bell peppers (from a 12-ounce jar), rinsed

- ¼ cup chopped fresh cilantro

- ¼ cup chopped toasted pistachios

Directions

- Step 1

Heat 1 tablespoon oil in a large nonstick or cast-iron skillet over medium-high heat. Pat salmon dry and sprinkle the flesh with 1/4 teaspoon each salt and pepper. Add to the pan, skin-side up, and cook until lightly browned, 3 to 4 minutes. Turn and cook until it's just cooked through and flakes easily with a fork, 1 to 2 minutes more. Transfer to a plate.

- Step 2

Meanwhile, whisk the remaining 2 tablespoons oil, 1/4 teaspoon each salt and pepper, vinegar and garlic in a medium bowl. Add quinoa, peppers, cilantro and pistachios; toss to combine. Serve the salmon with the salad.

Stuffed Potatoes with Salsa & Beans

Ingredients

- 4 medium russet potatoes

- ½ cup fresh salsa

- 1 ripe avocado, sliced

- 1 (15 ounce) can pinto beans, rinsed, warmed and lightly mashed

- 4 teaspoons chopped pickled jalapeños

Directions

- Step 1

Pierce potatoes all over with a fork. Microwave on Medium, turning once or twice, until soft, about 20 minutes. (Alternatively, bake potatoes at 425 degrees F until tender, 45 minutes to 1 hour.) Transfer to a clean cutting board and let cool slightly.

- Step 2

Holding them with a kitchen towel to protect your hands, make a lengthwise cut to open the potato, but don't cut all the way through. Pinch the ends to expose the flesh.

- Step 3

Top each potato with some salsa, avocado, beans and jalapeños. Serve warm.

Chickpea & Quinoa Grain Bowl

Ingredients

- 1 cup cooked quinoa

- ⅓ cup canned chickpeas, rinsed and drained

- ½ cup cucumber slices

- ½ cup cherry tomatoes, halved

- ¼ avocado, diced

- 3 tablespoons hummus

- 1 tablespoon finely chopped roasted red pepper

- 1 tablespoon lemon juice

- 1 tablespoon water, plus more if desired

- 1 teaspoon chopped fresh parsley (Optional)

- Pinch of salt

- Pinch of ground pepper

Directions

- Step 1

Arrange quinoa, chickpeas, cucumbers, tomatoes and avocado in a wide bowl.

• Step 2

Stir hummus, roasted red pepper, lemon juice and water in a bowl. Add more water to reach desired consistency for dressing. Add parsley, salt and pepper and stir to combine. Serve with the Buddha bowl.

Pistachio-&-Halloumi-Crusted Halibut

Ingredients

• ¼ cup shredded halloumi cheese

• ¼ cup finely chopped unsalted pistachios

• ¼ cup panko breadcrumbs

• 1 scallion, minced

• ½ teaspoon grated lemon zest, plus lemon wedges for serving

• 1 ¼ pounds halibut fillet, cut into 4 portions

- ¼ teaspoon ground pepper

- ⅛ teaspoon garlic salt

- 1 ½ tablespoons mayonnaise

Directions

- Step 1

Preheat oven to 400°F. Coat a baking sheet with cooking spray or line with foil.

- Step 2

Stir cheese, pistachios, panko, scallion and lemon zest in a small bowl. Place halibut on the prepared pan and sprinkle with pepper and garlic salt . Brush the top of the fish with mayonnaise, then coat with the pistachio mixture, pressing to help it adhere.

- Step 3

Bake until the fish is opaque and flakes easily with a fork, 8 to 12 minutes. Serve with lemon wedges, if desired.

Chicken & Vegetable Penne with Parsley-Walnut Pesto

Ingredients

- ¾ cup chopped walnuts

- 1 cup lightly packed parsley leaves

- 2 cloves garlic, crushed and peeled

- ½ teaspoon plus 1/8 teaspoon salt

- ⅛ teaspoon ground pepper

- 2 tablespoons olive oil

- ⅓ cup grated Parmesan cheese

- 1 ½ cups shredded or sliced cooked skinless chicken breast (8 oz.)

- 6 ounces whole-wheat penne or fusilli pasta (1 3/4 cups)

- 8 ounces green beans, trimmed and halved crosswise (2 cups)

- 2 cups cauliflower florets (8 oz.)

Directions

- Step 1

Bring a large pot of water to a boil.

- Step 2

Place walnuts in a small bowl and microwave on High until fragrant and lightly toasted, 2 to 2 1/2 minutes. (Alternatively, toast the walnuts in a small dry skillet over medium-low heat, stirring constantly, until fragrant, 2 to 3 minutes.) Transfer to a plate and let cool. Set 1/4 cup aside for topping.

- Step 3

Combine the remaining 1/2 cup walnuts, parsley, garlic, salt, and pepper in a food processor. Process until the nuts are ground. With the motor running, gradually add oil through the feed tube. Add Parmesan and pulse until mixed in. Scrape the pesto into a large bowl. Add chicken.

- Step 4

Meanwhile, cook pasta in the boiling water for 4 minutes. Add green beans and cauliflower; cover and cook until the pasta is al dente (almost tender) and the vegetables are tender, 5 to 7 minutes more. Before draining, scoop out 3/4 cup of the cooking water and stir it into the pesto-chicken mixture to warm it slightly. Drain the pasta and vegetables and add to the pesto-chicken mixture. Toss to coat well. Divide among 4 pasta bowls and top each serving with 1 Tbsp. of the reserved walnuts.

Poached Cod & Green Beans with Pesto

Ingredients

- 1 tablespoon extra-virgin olive oil

- 1 pound green and/or yellow wax beans, trimmed

- ¾ cup thinly sliced shallot

- 1 ¼ pounds cod (see Tip), cut into 4 portions

- ¼ teaspoon salt

- ¼ teaspoon freshly ground pepper

- 1 ½ cups low-sodium chicken broth or "no-chicken" broth

- ¼ cup prepared pesto

- Lemon wedges for serving

Directions

- Step 1

Heat oil in a large skillet over medium-high heat. Add beans and shallot and cook, stirring occasionally, until the shallot starts to soften, 1 to 2 minutes.

- Step 2

Sprinkle both sides of cod with salt and pepper. Spread the beans into a flat layer in the pan and gently place the cod on top. Increase heat to high, add broth, cover and cook until the fish is just cooked through, 4 to 6 minutes.

- Step 3

With a slotted spoon, transfer the cod and beans to a large serving plate or divide among 4 dinner plates;

cover to keep warm. Cook the broth over high heat, uncovered, until reduced to about 1/2 cup, about 5 minutes. Remove from heat and stir in pesto. Pour the sauce over the fish and beans and serve with lemon wedges, if desired.

Chickpea Coconut Curry

Ingredients

- 2 tablespoons extra-virgin olive oil

- 1 small white onion, finely diced

- 2 teaspoons minced fresh ginger

- 1 clove garlic, minced

- 2 teaspoons garam masala

- 1 teaspoon ground cumin

- ½ teaspoon ground coriander

- ¼ teaspoon salt plus a pinch, divided

- ¼ cup tomato paste

- 1 14-ounce can reduced-fat or light coconut milk (see Tip)

- 1 15-ounce can no-salt-added chickpeas, rinsed

- 1 tablespoon lemon juice

- Chopped fresh cilantro for garnish

Directions

- Step 1

Heat oil in a large saucepan over medium heat. Add onion and cook, stirring frequently, until soft and starting to brown, 3 to 4 minutes. Stir in ginger, garlic, garam masala, cumin, coriander and ¼ teaspoon salt; cook, stirring, for 1 minute. Add tomato paste and cook, stirring, for 30 seconds. Stir in coconut milk and bring to a simmer. Cook, stirring occasionally, until slightly thickened, about 5 minutes. Remove from heat.

- Step 2

Puree the sauce with an immersion blender or in a regular blender until smooth. (Use caution when pureeing hot liquids.) Return the sauce to the pot, if necessary, and add chickpeas, lemon juice and the remaining pinch of salt. Sprinkle with cilantro, if desired.

Chickpea Coconut Curry

Ingredients

- 2 tablespoons extra-virgin olive oil

- 1 small white onion, finely diced

- 2 teaspoons minced fresh ginger

- 1 clove garlic, minced

- 2 teaspoons garam masala

- 1 teaspoon ground cumin

- ½ teaspoon ground coriander

- ¼ teaspoon salt plus a pinch, divided

- ¼ cup tomato paste

- 1 14-ounce can reduced-fat or light coconut milk (see Tip)

- 1 15-ounce can no-salt-added chickpeas, rinsed

- 1 tablespoon lemon juice

- Chopped fresh cilantro for garnish

Directions

- Step 1

Heat oil in a large saucepan over medium heat. Add onion and cook, stirring frequently, until soft and starting to brown, 3 to 4 minutes. Stir in ginger, garlic, garam masala, cumin, coriander and ¼ teaspoon salt; cook, stirring, for 1 minute. Add tomato paste and cook, stirring, for 30 seconds. Stir in coconut milk and bring to a simmer. Cook, stirring occasionally, until slightly thickened, about 5 minutes. Remove from heat.

- Step 2

Puree the sauce with an immersion blender or in a regular blender until smooth. (Use caution when pureeing hot liquids.) Return the sauce to the pot, if necessary, and add chickpeas, lemon juice and the remaining pinch of salt. Sprinkle with cilantro, if desired.

Whole-Grain Spaghetti with Italian Turkey Sausage, Arugula & Balsamic Tomato Sauce

Ingredients

- 1 tablespoon olive oil

- 6 ounces sweet or hot Italian turkey sausage, casings removed

- 12 ounces cherry tomatoes or multicolor cherry tomatoes, halved if very large

- 1 cup chopped yellow onion

- 6 small garlic cloves, thinly sliced

- ¼ cup dry white wine

- 2 ½ cups unsalted chicken stock

- ½ teaspoon black pepper

- 8 ounces whole-grain spaghetti noodles, broken in half

- 5 ounces baby arugula

- 2 tablespoons red wine vinegar

- 2 tablespoons chopped fresh basil

- ¼ cup finely grated Parmesan cheese

Directions

- Step 1

Heat oil in a Dutch oven over medium-high. Add sausage, and cook, stirring often to break into pieces, until sausage is barely pink, about 4 minutes. Add tomatoes, onion, and garlic, and cook, stirring often, until vegetables are softened, about 4 more minutes. Add wine, and cook until reduced by half, about 2 minutes, scraping bottom of Dutch oven to release any browned bits. Add chicken stock and pepper, and bring to a boil. Add broken pasta, and stir, making sure pasta is mostly submerged. Reduce heat to medium; cover and cook until pasta is al dente, about 7 minutes.

- Step 2

Remove from heat, and stir in arugula and vinegar. Toss until arugula is wilted, about 1 minute. Spoon 1 1/2 cups into each of 4 bowls, and top each bowl with basil and 1 tablespoon of cheese.

SUMMARY

Alzheimer's is a complicated disease, and scientists are working on unlocking its secrets. Living a healthy lifestyle may help prevent it. If you have a family history of Alzheimer's, it's important to discuss it with your doctor.

By the time Alzheimer's is diagnosed, the progression of the disease can't be stopped. But treatment can help delay symptoms and improve your quality of life.

If you think you or a loved one may have Alzheimer's, talk with a doctor. They can help make a diagnosis, discuss what you can expect, and help connect you with services and support. If you're interested, they can also give you information about taking part in clinical trials.